Homemade Soaps:

100 % Organic and Natural Soaps With Step-by-Step Guide

Table of Content:

Introduction Soap—Common but Crucial

Soap is such a ubiquitous household item that we often find ourselves taking it for granted. But if we suddenly didn't have soap, we would rather quickly realize what we were missing. Besides not being hygienic and opening ourselves up to germs—not being clean could only lead to discomfort and low self-esteem. You see, we all take pride in our cleanliness whether we realize it or not.

If you don't believe this to be the case, just try stepping out of bed in the morning without taking a shower, without combing your hair, without wearing deodorant, and without brushing your teeth. You would feel kind of strange and uncomfortable, wouldn't you? Like you need to reach for a good bar of soap, right? Exactly! Because without soap we just don't feel like ourselves, and are not at our best.

There was a reason soap was invented some 5,000 odd years ago—because it makes us feel good. And you'll be feeling even better when you can create and alternate your very own varieties of soap as this book allows you to do. Yes, soap may indeed be common, but it is just as crucial today as when our cave man ancestors first cooked up a batch of lye. Because we all need soap in order to feel alright!

Chapter 1: Homemade Cleansers and Detoxifying Soap

Nothing feels better than a good facial cleanser. A good soap cleanser should be able to remove sediments from the skin and clear out abrasive oils. Detoxifying soap is also good at ridding the skin of harmful additives in order to bring back a more natural sheen. Here in this chapter you will find a wide variety of recipes for homemade cleansers and detoxifying soap.

Coconut Cleansing Soap

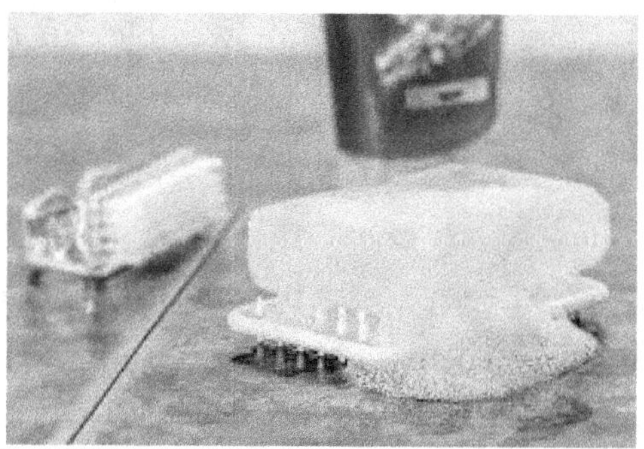

This type of soap is just perfect for cleansing away impurities from the skin. The silky-smooth coconut blend is so soothing that even the roughest of surfaces will soon be on the mend!

It's no joke. In this recipe coconut oil, palm oil, and castor oil came together to make an altogether unforgettable soap!

<u>Here are the exact ingredients:</u>

- ✓ *8 ounces of coconut oil*
- ✓ *8 ounces of palm oil*
- ✓ *15 ounces of castor oil*
- ✓ *2 cups of water*

To get started on this one, first take out a medium sized mixing bowl and add your 2 cups of water. After you have done this, you can then add your 8 ounces of coconut oil, and your 8 ounces of palm oil, followed by your 15 ounces of castor oil.

Once these ingredients are in place, mix them all together well and allow the mixing bowl to sit outside at room temperature a moment, so that it can all settle in place.

After it has all settled in well, you can then pour the blended ingredients into a set of prearranged soap molds. The soaps should become solid after about 10 hours. Once solid simply remove from the molds and they are ready for use.

Fruity Facial Soap

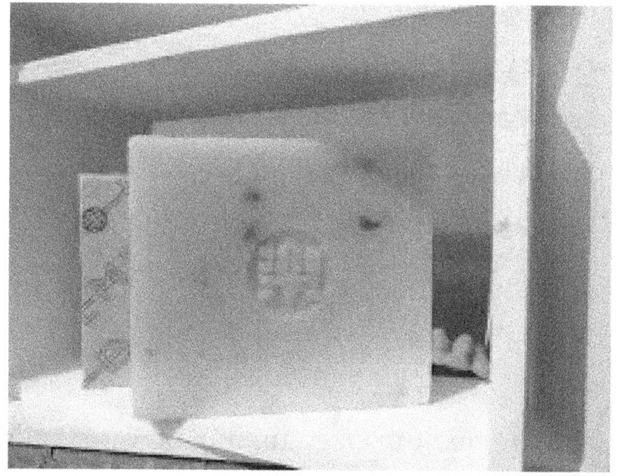

The name may of this soap blend may not exactly roll right off your tongue but it's a potent piece of soap work all the same! Decked out with olive oil, palm oil, coconut oil, lemon oil, and orange—this soap comes loaded for bear!

Fruity Facial Soap provides your skin with more nutrients and valuable minerals than money can buy. Sometimes our face could use a tropical blend of ingredients in order to make things just right! Go ahead and give this fruity facial soap a try!

<u>Here are the exact ingredients:</u>

- ✓ *5 ounces of olive oil*
- ✓ *3 ounces of palm oil*
- ✓ *10 ounces of coconut oil*
- ✓ *10 ounces of lemon oil*
- ✓ *10 ounces of orange oil*
- ✓ *2 ounces of lye*
- ✓ *2 cups of water*

First, take out a medium sized mixing bowl and add your 5 ounces of olive oil followed by your 3 ounces of palm oil, your 10 ounces of coconut oil, your 10 ounces of lemon oil, and your 10 ounces of orange oil. Vigorously stir all of these ingredients together until you have created a thoroughly blended mix.

Once you have done this, allow the ingredients to sit outside at room temperature so that they can congeal together. Next, add in your 2 ounces of lye followed by your 2 cups of water. Finally, mix everything together and pour mixture into your soap molds. After about 8 to 10 hours the soaps should become solid. Once solid, simply take them out of the molds and use when ready.

Citrus Soap Detox

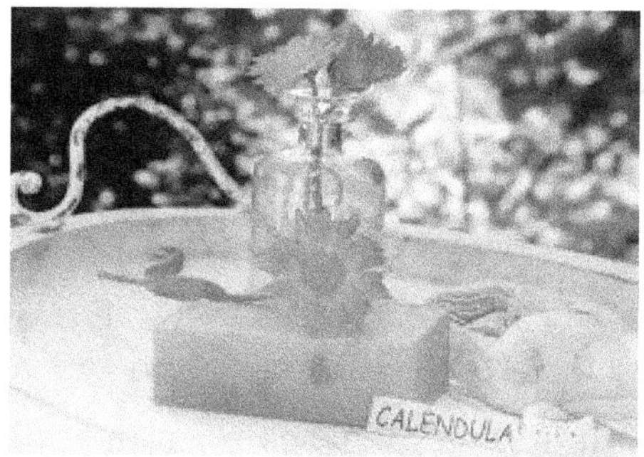

Citrus based fruits serve as a natural cleansing agent. It is for this reason that so many over the counter cleaners have lemon and other citrus ingredients in them. Lemon is great at knocking away tough stains and odors. But citrus oils can do more than just scrub away at our dishes, sinks, and counters.

These essential oils are also quite good for your health as antioxidants and immune boosting disinfectants. And as this Citrus Detox Soap can testify—they provide a powerful form of detox for our skin. When it comes to our personal hygiene and health sometimes, we have to think a little bit outside the box. So, do yourself a favor and try this Citrus Soap Detox!

<u>Here are the exact ingredients:</u>

- ✓ *10 drops of lemon oil*
- ✓ *10 drops of orange oil*
- ✓ *3 ounces of lye*
- ✓ *2 cups of water*

Get out a medium sized mixing bowl and add your 10 drops of lemon oil and your 10 drops of orange oil. Stir these together briefly before dumping in your 2 cups of water followed by your 3 ounces of lye. Now stir it all together well and allow to sit out at room temperature a moment so that everything settles in place.

Once you have done this, pour your soap mixture into your soap molds and allow everything to solidify and harden over the course of the next 10 hours. After this, your soaps are ready for use.

Hot Cocoa Butter Soap

Everybody likes hot cocoa and everybody hopefully likes soap. So, what about some Hot Cocoa Butter Soap?

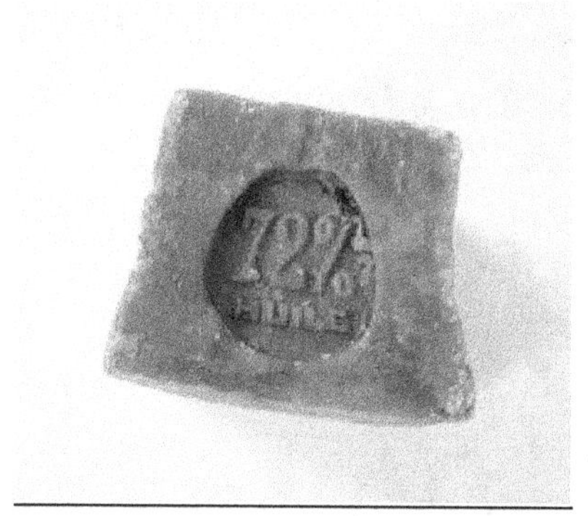

The name is actually a bit of a misnomer because the hotness of this soap comes not from hot chocolate, but spicy hot habenero peppers! Yes, incredibly enough, a blend of habenero and cocoa butter is just what the doctor ordered when it comes to having an effective cleanser! If you would like to give your skin a warm glow, give this recipe a go!

<u>Here are the exact ingredients:</u>

- ✓ *3 ounces of habenero oil*
- ✓ *10 ounces of coconut oil*
- ✓ *10 ounces of castor oil*
- ✓ *10 ounces of avocado oil*
- ✓ *5 ounces of mango butter*
- ✓ *5 ounces of cocoa butter*
- ✓ *3 ounces of lye*
- ✓ *2 cups of water*

Take out a small container or mixing bowl and add your 3 ounces of habenero oil followed by your 10 ounces of coconut oil, your 10 ounces of castor oil, your 10 ounces of avocado oil, your 5 ounces of cocoa butter, and your 5 ounces of mango butter.

Now stir, or even simply swirl the ingredients together with your hand. After this go ahead and add in your 3 ounces of lye, and your 2 cups of water. Stir everything together well, and then pour the mixed ingredients into your soap molds. Give them about 8 hours to solidify and use when ready.

Banana Hydration Soap

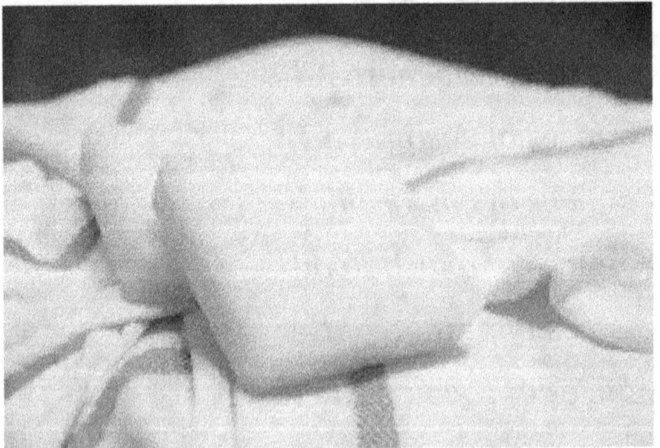

At any given time, we could be suffering from some sort of nutrient deficiency. In fact, just about any given ailment of the body is usually quite easily solved when certain depleted resources are replenished. And one of those certain resources is potassium.

The Banana has naturally fortifying and hydrating ingredients such as potassium that can completely restore dry and cracked skin. If this sounds like something you might need, then by all means, try this recipe out for yourself.

<u>Here are the exact ingredients:</u>

- ✓ *10 drops of banana oil*
- ✓ *5 ounces of canola oil*
- ✓ *5 ounces of vegetable oil*
- ✓ *2 tablespoons of sugar*
- ✓ *5 ounces of lye*
- ✓ *3 cups of water*

Just get out a medium sized mixing bowl and add your 10 drops of banana oil followed by your 5 ounces of canola oil, and your 5 ounces of vegetable oil.

Stir all of these ingredients together well before adding in your 2 tablespoons of sugar. Stir one more time and allow to settle at room temperature. After this add your 5 ounces of lye and your 3 cups of water. Now stir everything together one final time before pouring the mixture into your soap molds. Allow to solidify for about 12 hours and your soap is ready for use.

Iodine Detox Soap

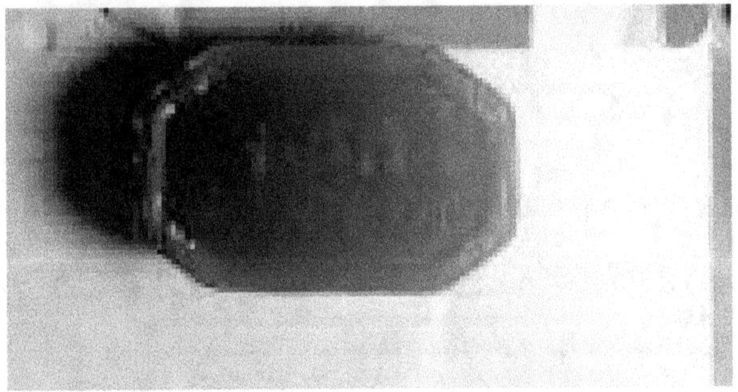

Did you ever scrape your knee as a kid and have someone put iodine on the wound? There is a reason for this. Iodine is a wonderful cleansing and detoxifying agent. It helps to speed up the healing process even as it disinfects. And when compressed into a bar of soap it can really do some wonders.

Whether you have cuts and scrapes, or simply need a little bit of extra healing, Iodine Detox Soap is a great resource to have on hand. If you need an extra boost just lather yourself up in the healing and rejuvenating powers of Iodine Detox Soap! Try this recipe and find out for yourself!

<u>Here are the exact ingredients:</u>

- ✓ *5 ounces of iodine*
- ✓ *5 ounces of olive oil*
- ✓ *3 ounces of milk*
- ✓ *2 ounces of lye*
- ✓ *2 cups of water*

First, get out a medium sized container or mixing bowl and add your 5 ounces of iodine, and your 5 ounces of olive oil. Mix all of these ingredients together well before adding in your 3 ounces of milk, your 2 ounces of lye, and your 2 cups of water.

Stir everything together well and pour into your soap molds. Allow the soaps to solidify and harden over the course of the next 7 to 8 hours. Once solid, take out of the molds and use when ready.

Chapter 2: Essential Oil Organic Soap

Essential oils have long been a part of various forms of holistic medicine such as aromatherapy and massage therapy for quite some time. So, it only makes sense that many benefits can be gleaned from soaps which use these powerful ingredients. Browse through some of the recipes presented in this chapter and see for yourself!

Lavender Essential Oil Soap

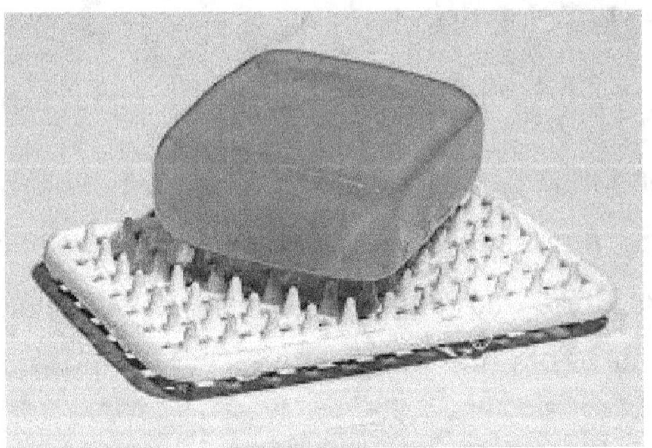

It seems that almost all of the bodily senses are consoled by a dose of lavender. Lavender is soothing to the eye, nose, and touch—and if it could speak up and talk to us, its voice would probably soothe us as well!

Not many elements can come close to the calming serenity of this essential oil. And when placed in a bar of soap, these attributes become even more enhanced. If you need to allow your skin the chance to relax, Lavender Essential Oil Soap might be just what the doctor ordered.

<u>Here are the exact ingredients:</u>

- ✓ *10 tablespoons of lavender oil*
- ✓ *5 tablespoons of coconut oil*
- ✓ *5 tablespoons of olive oil*
- ✓ *5 tablespoons of palm oil*
- ✓ *5 tablespoons of almond oil*
- ✓ *2 cups of water*

Get out a medium sized mixing bowl and add your 10 tablespoons of lavender oil followed by your 5 tablespoons of coconut oil, your 5 tablespoons of olive oil, your 5 tablespoons of palm oil, and your 5 tablespoons of almond oil. Follow this up by adding in your 2 cups of water. Stir everything together well and pour into your soap molds. The soaps should become solid after 5 to 7 hours. Use when ready.

Almond Essential Oil Soap

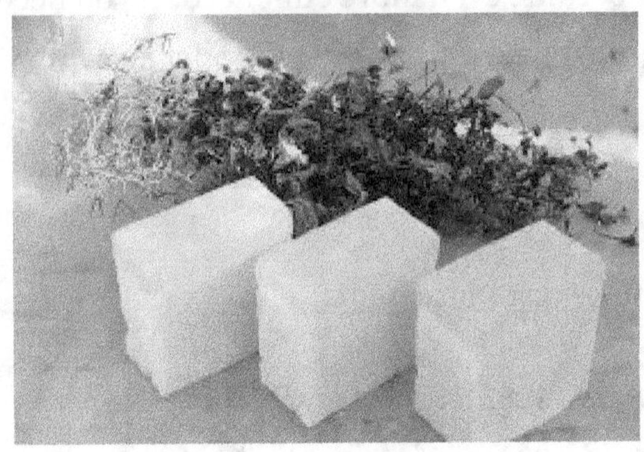

Soap made of essential almond oil should be a part of your essential routine! Almond essential oil has powerful antioxidants that help to exfoliate the skin even as it cleanses the dirt and grime away. This soap has the ability to clean and cleanse like no other! Go ahead and make your own today!

<u>Here are the exact ingredients:</u>

- ✓ 20 ounces of soybean oil
- ✓ 10 ounces of palm oil
- ✓ 8 ounces of coconut oil
- ✓ 4 ounces of almond oil
- ✓ 2 cups of water

Add your 20 ounces of soybean oil, followed by your 10 ounces of palm oil, your 8 ounces of coconut oil, and your 4 ounces of almond oil into a medium sized mixing bowl or container. After this, add your 2 cups of water and stir the ingredients together well.

Allow to sit out room temperature for a minute or two until the structure has congealed and settled thoroughly. After this, pour the mixture into your soap molds, allow to solidify over the next 8 to 10 hours and you are good to go!

Peppermint Essential Soap

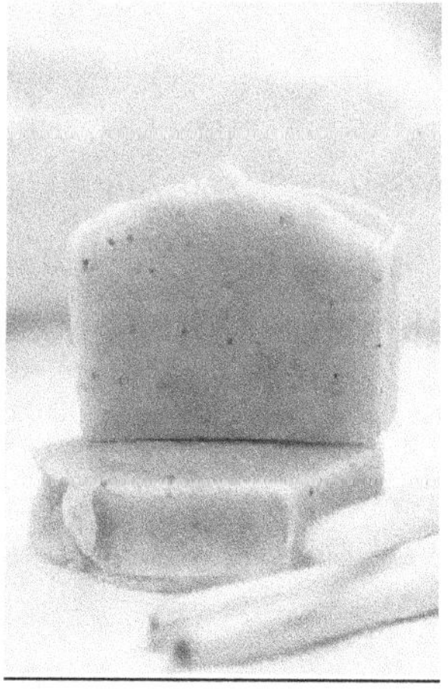

Peppermint essential oil is good for a lot of different things and smooth, clean skin is one of them! Peppermint is also a known immune booster and helps to rejuvenate aching muscles and joints! You really need to take some stock of your health, so try out this Peppermint Essential Oil Soap for yourself

<u>Here are the exact ingredients:</u>

- ✓ *5 ounces of coconut oil*
- ✓ *4 ounces of palm oil*
- ✓ *7 ounces of peppermint oil*
- ✓ *6 drops of grapefruit seed extract*
- ✓ *4 ounces of lye*
- ✓ *2 cups of water*

With a mixing bowl handy, go ahead and add in your 5 ounces of coconut oil, 4 ounces of palm oil, and 7 ounces of peppermint oil. Stir these ingredients together well and allow them to settle and congeal at room temperature for a moment. Next, add in your 4 ounces of lye and your 2 cups of water.

Stir these ingredients together well for 1 to 2 minutes. Once thoroughly stirred, pour the entire mixture into your soap molds. Allow to harden in the molds for at least 8 hours. After this, the soap should be ready for use.

Lemon Essential Oil Soap

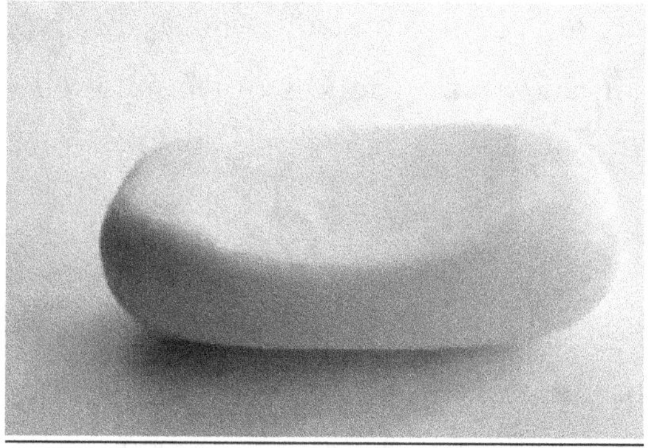

Whether it's the lemon scented dish soap on your kitchen counter or the lemon scented air freshener hanging from the rearview mirror of your car—lemon is everywhere when it comes to things that are fresh and clean. Lemon washes the grime and dirt away like no other. So, if you are in need of a heavy-duty cleanser this recipe is highly recommended.

<u>Here are the exact ingredients:</u>

- ✓ *10 drops of lemon essential oil*
- ✓ *3 drops of orange essential oil*
- ✓ *4 ounces of lye*
- ✓ *2 cups of water*

Take out a small to medium sized mixing bowl and add your 10 drops of lemon essential oil, your 3 drops of orange essential oil, and your 4 ounces of lye followed by your 2 cups of water.

Stir everything together well and set to the side to settle for a couple of minutes. After this pour the mixture into your soap molds and allow to harden over the next 10 hours. Once they have properly solidified just pope them out of the molds and they are ready for use.

Clove Essential Oil Soap

Clove essential oil provides us with a boost of healthy and heartening rejuvenation. This powerful essential oil is proven to boost the immune system and curtail infection.

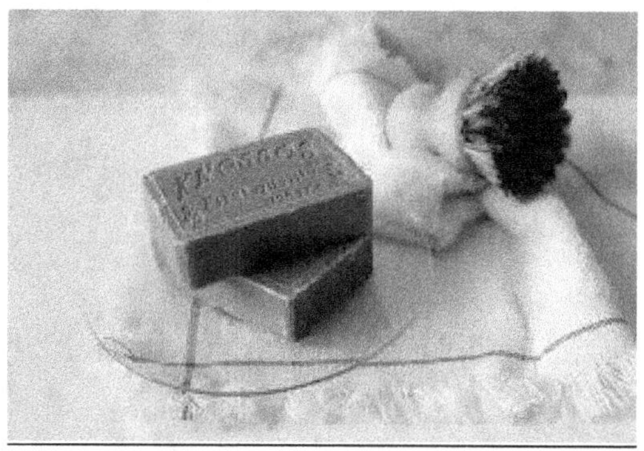

This is a great asset when it comes to recovering from sickness or injury. Add this fantastic recipe to your soap inventory and you will have something that's good for just about anything that may be ailing you! Give Clove Essential Oil Soap a try!

<u>Here are the exact ingredients:</u>

- ✓ *10 drops of clove essential oil*
- ✓ *5 drops of rose essential oil*
- ✓ *2 ounces of lye*
- ✓ *1 cup of water*

In a small mixing bowl or container, add your 10 drops of clove essential oil, and your 5 drops of rose essential oil. Stir the ingredients or even swirl them together in your hand.

Once they are mixed together go ahead and add your 2 ounces of lye and your cup of water. Mix all of these ingredients together as thoroughly as possible before dumping the mixture into your soap molds.

Once inside the molds allow to harden and solidify over the course of the next 10 hours. Once solid, break the soaps out of their molds and use when ready.

Chapter 3: Organic Soap for Your Daily Routine

Organic soap is more than just a trend—it's a way of life. Because being able to use soap that is free from all the harmful chemicals and additives that are found in store bought varieties is truly a life changing experience. Here in this chapter you will find several great organic soap recipes to fit your routine.

Shaving Cream Soap

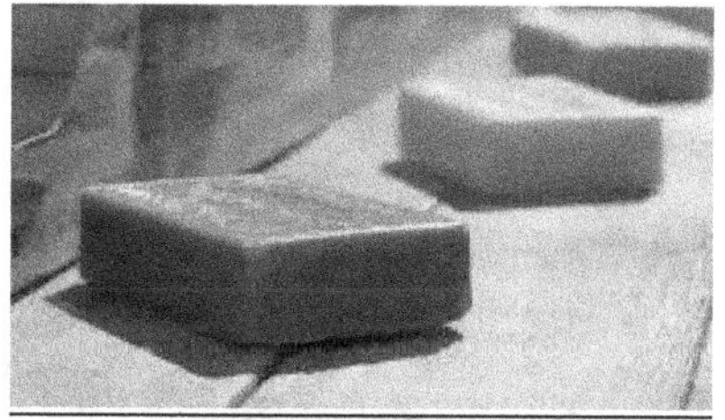

Are you in need of a good soapy shave? Do you need a cream that will last and with a consistency that will not fade? Well, this soap's shelf life is good—whether you need to shave your face or your legs—this soap does the job like no one else could! So, don't delay! Try this Shaving Cream Soap out for yourself today!

<u>Here are the exact ingredients:</u>

- ✓   *15 ounces of coconut oil*
- ✓   *10 ounces of olive oil*
- ✓   *10 ounces of palm oil*
- ✓   *5 ounces of buttermilk*
- ✓   *4 ounces of lye*
- ✓   *2 cups of water*

Get out a medium sized mixing bowl and add your 15 ounces of coconut oil, your 10 ounces of olive oil, your 10 ounces of palm oil, your 5 ounces of buttermilk, your 4 ounces of lye and your 2 cups of water. Stir the ingredients together well and allow to settle for a moment.

Once settled pour the mixture into your soap molds and leave to harden over the course of the next 8 to 10 hours. Once solidified, break the soaps out of their molds and use when ready.

Organic B.O. Busting Soap

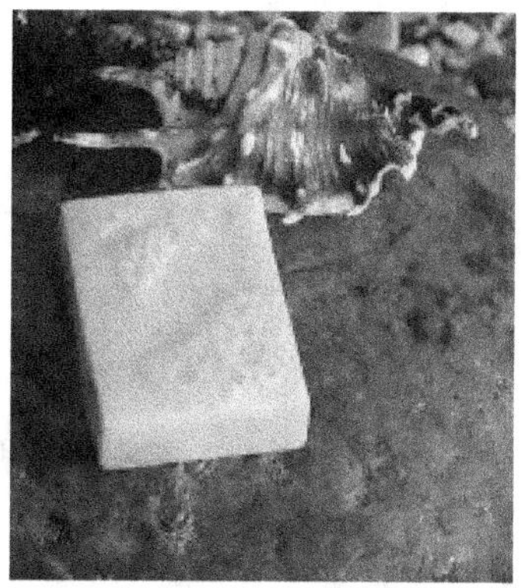

It may be embarrassing, but it's a fact of life. We get warm, we sweat, and we produce body odor. Having that said, the last thing any of us needs is to walk into the room and be the center of bad B.O. attention. But sometimes our regular deodorant either just isn't powerful enough to mask odor, or it simply produces too frustrating side effects.

Some deodorants in fact, can quickly become skin irritants, and in some cases, can even lead to acute allergic reactions. So, what is going to help? What is one to do? Well, just keep reading folks, because this Organic B.O. Busting Soap is for you!

<u>Here are the exact ingredients:</u>

- ✓ *10 ounces of olive oil*
- ✓ *5 ounces of beeswax*
- ✓ *5 drops of Ylang Ylang*
- ✓ *5 drops of Frankincense oil*

Inside a medium sized container add your 10 ounces of olive oil, followed by your 5 drops of Ylang Ylang, your 5 drops of Frankincense oil, and your 5 ounces of beeswax. Stir everything together well and allow to settle for a moment at room temperature. After a moment come back to the ingredients and pour them into your soap molds. Allow them to solidify within the molds for at least 7 hours before use.

Shampoo and Body Wash Soap

What do we have here my friends? Oh, my gosh! Here is a two in one blast of goodness—because these soapy suds provide you with both shampoo and body wash! You've just got to give this recipe a try!

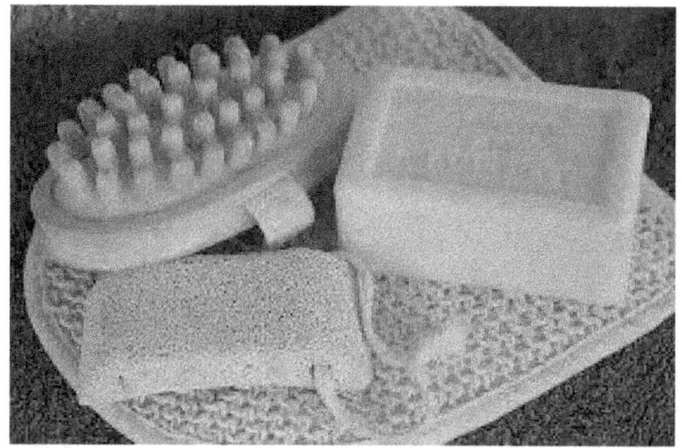

Here are the exact ingredients:

- ✓ 10 drops of coconut oil
- ✓ 8 drops of frankincense oil
- ✓ 8 drops of lavender oil
- ✓ 6 drops of jasmine oil
- ✓ 10 drops of lemon oil
- ✓ 5 drops of cocoa butter
- ✓ 4 ounces of lye
- ✓ 3 cups of water

Get out a large mixing bowl and add your 10 drops of coconut oil, your 8 drops of frankincense oil, your 8 drops of lavender oil, your 6 drops of jasmine oil, your 10 drops of lemon oil, and your 5 drops of cocoa butter.

After you have done this, you can then go ahead and add in your 4 ounces of lye and your 3 cups of water. Stir everything together well and allow to settle in at room temperature for about 2 minutes.

Once everything is nicely settled and congealed together, pour the mixture into your soap molds. Once poured into the molds, allow the mixture to solidify over the course of the next 10 hours. Once the soaps have hardened sufficiently, they are ready to use. Enjoy!

Milk and Honey Soap

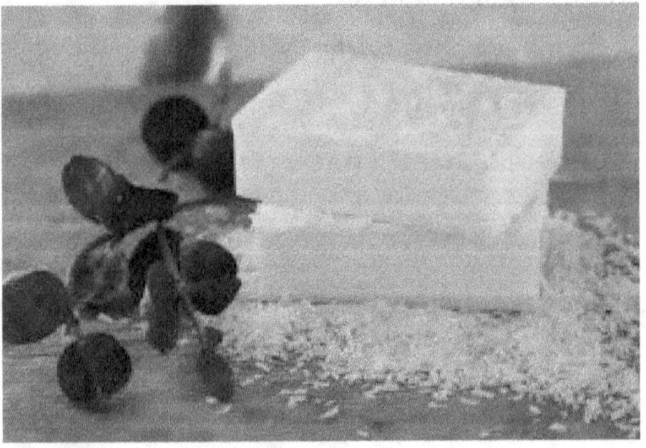

Nothing goes together quite like milk and honey and when they are coupled together to create a good bar of soap—the results are absolutely fantastic. The consistency of coconut, gives you an epidermal layer that is even and balanced.

The soap melts right into your skin as it lathers, automatically giving you a nice and shiny sheen. If you are looking for a good clean and soft skin to go with it, Milk and Honey Soap gets the job done quite nicely.

<u>Here are the exact ingredients:</u>

- ✓ *12 ounces of honey*
- ✓ *5 ounces of coconut oil*
- ✓ *3 ounces of milk*
- ✓ *2 ounces of lye*
- ✓ *2 cups of water*

For this one, get out a medium sized mixing bowl and add your 12 ounces of honey, your 5 ounces of coconut oil, your 3 ounces of milk, followed by your 2 ounces of lye and 2 cups of water. Stir everything together well and allow to settle at room temperature for about 3 minutes

After this, pour the mixture into soap molds and let them harden for 10 hours. Once solidified simply break the soaps out of their molds and get ready to use them!

Morning Coconut Soap

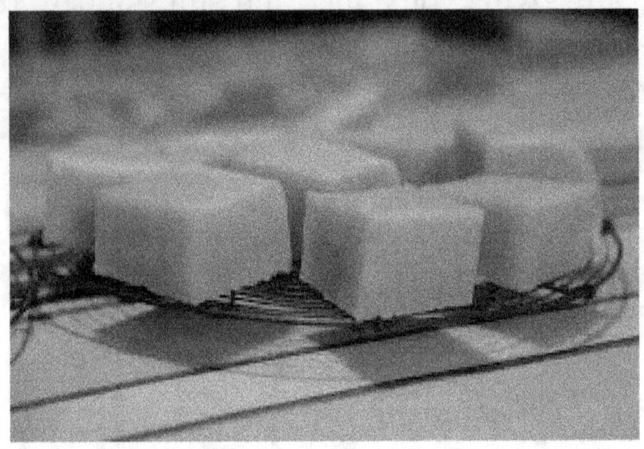

Nothing beats Morning Coconut Soap. My oh—my oh my! There are no ifs, ands, or buts. If you like the idea of waking up to soothing coconut—give this soap a try!

<u>Here are the exact ingredients:</u>

- ✓ *12 ounces of coconut oil*
- ✓ *8 ounces of olive oil*

- ✓   *6 ounces of castor oil*
- ✓   *4 ounces of rose oil*
- ✓   *3 ounces of lye*
- ✓   *4 cups of water*

In a large container or mixing bowl add your 12 ounces of coconut oil, your 8 ounces of olive oil, your 6 ounces of castor oil, your 4 ounces of rose oil, your 3 ounces of lye, followed by your 4 cups of water.

Now mix everything together well and sit the container out to settle at room temperature. Once settled, pour ingredients into your individual soap molds and allow to harden. For this type of soap, you should allow at least 12 hours for your soaps to fully harden before use.

Chapter 4: Rare and Unique Soap Blends

As we bring this book to its conclusion, I would like to inundate you with one last chapter that showcases some of the more rare and unique blends of soap. These soaps are somewhat odd, and somewhat funny but even so, they still have essential value when it comes to your personal needs. Just think of it as soap with a twist! At any rate, here are some soap recipes certain to raise some eyebrows!

Wacky Tabasco Soap

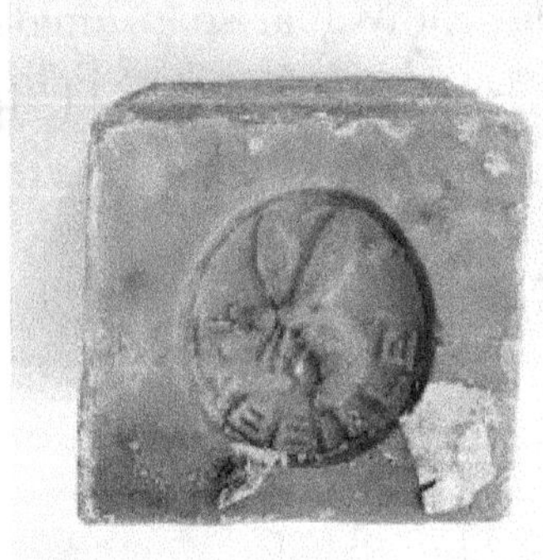

Really? Wacky Tabaco Soap? No! Read that again my friends, because this is Wacky Tabasco Soap! Its strange, its unique, and its kind of frightening, but believe it or not this soap can be downright enlightening!

Why is that? Because this Wacky Tabasco Soap is good for the complexion and smooths out skin that cracks! If you need for your skin to be restored to its original luster—Wacky Tabasco Soap is more than up for the task!

<u>Here are the exact ingredients:</u>

- ✓ *3 drops of tabasco sauce*
- ✓ *8 drops of coconut oil*
- ✓ *3 drops of buttermilk*
- ✓ *4 ounces of lye*
- ✓ *1 cup of water*

Inside a small to medium container add your 3 drops of tabasco sauce, your 8 drops of coconut oil, and your 3 drops of buttermilk. Stir these together well before leaving your mix out to settle for a few minutes. After this, go ahead and add your 4 ounces of lye and your cup of water.

Now just stir this potent blend together until it is all thoroughly mixed together. Once mixed, pour into your soap molds and allow to solidify for about 10 hours. Once hardened, take the soaps out of their individual soap molds and use when ready.

Organic Beer Bar

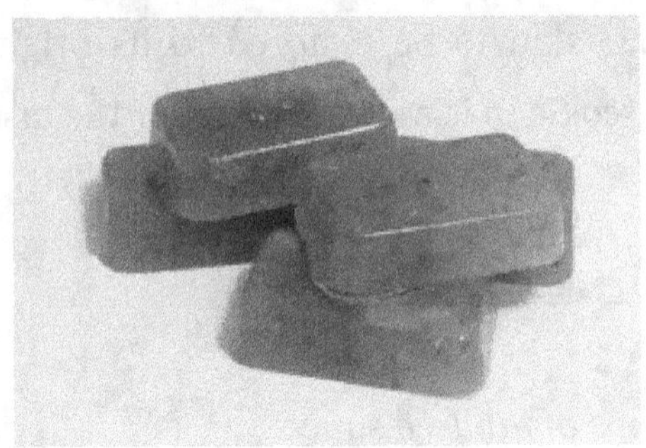

What's this? Is someone planning a beer bubble bath? No question about it. This is indeed quite an interesting piece of soap we've got here! And while no one is advocating getting a buzz from your bathwater, this completely Organic Beer Bar will make for a good bath all the same!

With 25 full ounces of beer infused with coconut and olive oil, this beer is strong and soothing. Don't hesitate to try it out for yourself!

<u>Here are the exact ingredients:</u>

- ✓ *25 ounces of beer (any kind)*
- ✓ *15 ounces of coconut oil*

- ✓ *15 ounces of olive oil*
- ✓ *5 ounces of lye*
- ✓ *2 cups of water*

Add your 25 ounces of beer, your 15 ounces of coconut oil, and your 15 ounces of olive oil to a large mixing bowl and stir the ingredients together. After this put the bowl in the refrigerator and allow ingredients to settle within the fridge for about a half hour.

Once a half hour has passed take the mixing bowl of ingredients out and deposit your 5 ounces of lye and 2 cups of water. Stir everything together well before pouring the entire mixture into your soap molds. Allow mix to sit within the soap molds for at least 8 hours. Once the soaps have hardened, they are ready for use.

Coca-Cola Suds Soap

Soda in your soap? Why not? All you need is a cup of Coca-Cola and a cup of lime juice and you are ready to go. If you are feeling down and out these soapy suds could lift your faltering spirits.

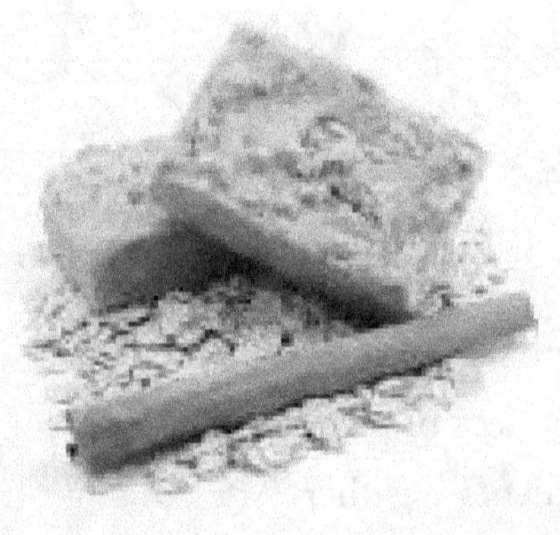

So, don't sit around and mope! If you are looking for a real pick me up—you've just got to try this Coca-Cola Suds Soap!

<u>Here are the exact ingredients:</u>

- ✓ *1 cup of Coca-Cola*
- ✓ *1 cup of lime juice*
- ✓ *4 ounces of lye*
- ✓ *2 cups of water*

Get out your medium sized mixing bowl and add your cup of Coca-Cola followed by your cup of lime juice. Stir these ingredients briefly before adding your 4 ounces of lye and two cups of water.

Now allow the ingredients to settle for just a moment before pouring them into your soap molds. Once they have hardened sufficiently, they should be good to go.

Creamy Chocolate Soap

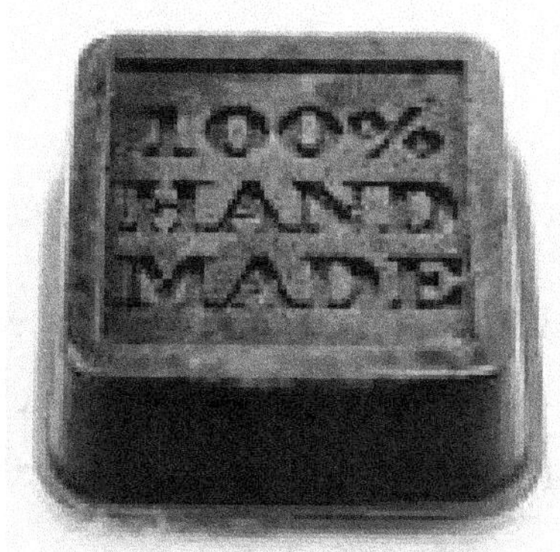

Do you like chocolate? Who doesn't like a chocolate fix every once in a while, right? Well, my friends—don't look far! With this recipe you can lather yourself up like you're a candy bar! What an ingenious blend of cocoa powder, cocoa butter and lye! Do yourself a favor and give this Creamy Chocolate Soap a try!

<u>Here are the exact ingredients:</u>

- ✓ *½ cup of cocoa powder*
- ✓ *4 drops of chocolate fragrance oil*
- ✓ *8 ounces of cocoa butter*
- ✓ *3 ounces of lye*
- ✓ *2 cups of water*

Deposit your ½ cup of cocoa powder, your 4 drops of chocolate fragrance oil, and your 8 ounces of cocoa butter into a medium sized mixing bowl. After you have done this place your 3 ounces of lye and 2 cups of water into the bowl as well. Stir everything well and allow to settle in place at room temperature for about a minute or two.

Finally, pour the mixture into your soap molds and allow them to solidify over the course of the next 10 hours. Once solid, just pop them out of your soap molds and they are ready for you to use.

Conclusion: We Could All Use Some Good Soap!

Soap is a vital necessity. Most of us wake up to a fresh lather of soap in the morning and our day wouldn't feel complete without it. But having that said, we need to be careful when it comes to the kinds of soap we are using since some of the store-bought varieties contain chemicals and other additives that could be harmful for our health.

This book offers a powerful alternative through a wide variety of DIY organic soap recipes. We could all use some good soap. So, just follow the instructions presented in this guide and you will have all the quality soap you could ever use!